God Does Not Hate Gays and Lesbians

...And Neither Should We!

God Does Not Hate Gays and Lesbians

...And Neither Should We!

Callie Carol Rodgers Jones

Printed in the United States of America

Editor: LPW Editing & Consulting Services, LLC

Cover Design: Mr. Daranta Levon Parker

First Printing, 2018

ISBN-13: 9781731083579

Scripture quotations are taken from the Holy Bible, King James Translation unless otherwise quoted.

Ordering Information: Books may be purchased in quantity and/or special sales by contacting Callie at calliescall55@gmail.com.

ALSO BY CALLIE CAROL RODGERS JONES

A Whale on Dry Land

Sweet Potato Pie

A Good Cry

Dedication

I dedicate this book to all of you who have and are suffering under the pain of abuse inflicted upon you through savage cruel people and years of feeling lost. God loves you and so do I. I encourage you to start your new life as God heals you of all the wounds that have left scars so undeserving.

Table of Contents

Acknowledgements......................................1

Chapter I: Understanding/Dealing with Issues......3

Chapter II: God's Intentions 15

Chapter III: Criminal Acts 23

Chapter IV: Be Ye Holy, Even as I am Holy.......33

Scripture References 37

Meet The Author....................................39

Acknowledgements

I would like to thank God, His Son Jesus and the precious Holy Spirit for leading and guiding me to write this book for the sole purpose of getting His message out about His love.

Special thanks to Mrs. Lita P. Ward of LPW Editing & Consulting Services, LLC for taking the time to edit my book. She is a blessing and a jewel. I also would like to thank my son Michael Jones for his contributions of getting me over my writer's block.

And last but not least, a heartfelt 'thank you" to my beloved husband, Bishop Jack H. Jones. He has been the one to encourage me the most. Thank you for your love and encouragement. I love you now, forever, for always.

Chapter I

Understanding and Dealing
With the Issues

Many people have issues against the question of this matter as to whether or not it is true or not. But the answer is written in God's Word. God, help your people! Much controversy has covered the land over men and women having same sex marriages. We have heard and seen these debates on social media, church gatherings, preachers preaching, etc. I recall in my younger days, seeing and hearing pieces of talk on these debates. But the issues I have seen and heard back then do not stand as intense as they are today. As a child I observed such happenings going on but it wasn't until eighth grade, when I was faced with the conversation of students I knew engaged in such acts. These were eighth graders saying what they would do because it involved fifty dollars. This was shocking for me to hear how young boys were engaging in some things of this nature! Moreover, it troubled me of how they made little of their actions because I knew they had girlfriends, who are dead today. From their deeds of committing these acts of anus play with other men, it only brought them diseases. And in turn, they brought those sicknesses back to their girlfriends and who would have become their future wives.

"These acts," the Bible calls them, have been a part of our world since the day after the fall of Adam, especially during the days of Sodom and Gomorrah, and it is like a running sore to our God's eyes. God's attention was brought on by the cries He heard from those that suffered death and abuse, and their blood cried out to Him from the grave. Just as the cry of

Abel, Cain's brother, whose voice cried out to God from the grave, after Cain took Abel's life. Most abusers know the pain they force on children and adults which causes their victims to feel lifeless. God cursed Cain for his selfish and evil act. This is found in the book of Genesis 4:10-11…

> *"And he said, what hast thou done? The voice of thy brother crieth unto me from the ground. And now art thou cursed from the earth, which hath opened her mouth to receive thy brother's blood from thy hand."*

Some never recover from such a grave experience. The Bible called the things that people did and do with their own gender wicked acts (abominations), inordinate affection, lasciviousness, carnalities acts. He sent His Son to heal so that He wouldn't have to look at the abominations in this world, and to keep His people from being hurt in this world. And as the Bible says, "To keep us from evil!" … from being destroyed by the work that comes at the mind. God desires those things to not have havoc with our thoughts, and cause

us to be a part of what the devil offers the world, which only

brings death and damnation to the soul.

Where did these things initiate? From the days of Adam,

disobedience or defiance of God is when these happenings of

rebellion began. As was then, the Bible says, *"Thou shalt*

not," but many question the reasoning of being told what not

to do. Why? Let us take a look back in the days when the

people of Israel went into the land of Egypt. During those

days the parents still taught the love and fear of God. And

they were reminded of whom to serve, that they would not be

influenced by other nationalities, which would pull them into

idol worshipping, witchcraft, worshipping of stars, the sun

and the moon; and yes the spirit of laying with animals and

being with their own gender. But slowly after those parents

died out, the teaching of right and wrong died also, as it is today! The true teaching of God's Word is not followed through as it should be today. You have false leaders abusing children while hiding behind the cloth. And with all that's going on, how come parents aren't being watchful? What a serious question to be asked! There are good parents who were careful but they trusted the wrong people to care for their children. And even in that situation, it's hurtful. But you can't blame yourself for all your children's pain unless you just don't or didn't care.

Because of the lack of nurturing and real love in homes, disobedient has streamed in the heart of so many children. When not being guarded, they become wicked people, which in turn, some of them will hurt and abuse those who are being left unattended. So when bad things happen, many want to charge God for it. He gave us these children to love and care for, not to allow others to destroy their lives through abuse which terminate the mind of all of its planned existence, placing them into a physical, spiritual, and mental state of being. Children can become prey in the hands of those who touched them; raped, abused or molested by family members, dads, boyfriends/girlfriends or even their own parents. Ninety-nine percent of these acts can originate from the assaulters, having been the assaulted. Some give themselves into these acts through trade. Someone will offer them things that they think could make their life better, such as fame or money. These don't realize that giving up their body to such acts will cause them to hate themselves in their future. Look at the suicide cases. Even after many have gotten older, but still in their minds, there is no peace. It does not matter how much money one can have or the friends who surround them, that peace of mind is the main source that keeps us holding on. One of the reasons so many people commit suicide is because they are being abused and they are abusing others. It is also another reason for many addicts using drugs and alcohol trying to end their pain. Suicide is not the answer to anyone's problems. The only way to end the pain is to find peace, not through the substitutes and destructions of this world, but by the peace of God through His Son Jesus. Philippians 2:5 says, *"Let this mind be in you, which was also in Christ Jesus."*

For the most, many are being taught that God does not exist. There are many parents who are church goers, and profess that they love God, but do not have enough love for their children to help heal their broken lives. While leaving them in the care of churchgoers, children are being raped by other boys, girls, men and women. And yes, when some children tell their parents and church about the forced abuse, the children are stoned mentally; by the ones they trusted (parents/church) to save them from their culprit. And instead of reporting the crime to the authorities, the church and parents want to keep it hush-hush, but God has a way of cleaning house.

A lot of parents don't find out that their child or children have gone through so much because the victim can be too afraid to tell what happened to them, or the minor may have been threatened by the offender. We hear stories of how teenagers and the elderly are being abuse in group homes, and even homes that Social Services have placed them in. I have had dreams of police officials taking children to an out of the way house, having pictures taken of children while they were naked, and some having sex with them. In my dream, the parents trusted these law enforcement officers, but the parents didn't know of the filthy acts that were taking place. Also in my dream, that sexual abuse was happening in a mental institution, abuse by the caregivers, while those that ran the facility knew about the things that went on, but chose to ignore it.

The problems also take place in schools, dorms, and other places where there isn't a sharp eye. It has been a while since I had this dream, but I saw in my sleep a young student that had just left home for college. She made friends with another student, who had been in college a while. This person was more like a senior in college. She knew her way around and she knew a lot of guys in that college as well. The senior was evil but that young student didn't know that. She really thought the older person was her friend. The young student was innocent and didn't know a lot about life. Her best friend was her mom. The young girl was invited to a party which was being held at the older girl's house. The young lady was excited and just smiled to even be with her older friend. Well, in walked a lot of guy friends and not one girl student was with them. One of them gave the senior a pernicious look, and that's when the senior gave the young student something to drink, but the young student didn't know she had spiked the punch. I could see the evilness in that senior but that poor child couldn't. After she drank the punch, she passed out. Then the senior nodded at the guys that were at the party; an indication that it was okay to have sex with the young girl.

The young girl later woke up feeling strange but she didn't understand why. Though she felt invaded, she still did not understand what had happened to her. Her mother was worrying about her because she was all she had and it was a while since she had heard from her baby. Her daughter was a good distance from her and she wanted to call her mom but because of the way she felt, she didn't know what to say. I share these dreams because I know that the things God shows me is happening and this is my way to warn people because I care.

People with evil hearts and wicked minds will force the innocent to literally seclude their life from people because they have been made to feel like nothing. The end results for them is to turn to what makes them feel comfortable, even though they don't see it as wrong, and it is, but this is their way of saying this is how it is. I have to tell you that many have lost their innocence through force and was a victim of evil beings; this is not how it should be or was ever meant to be. God never intended for life to be this way. Those that hurt you then are no longer the ones that are hurting you; it is you that's doing the inflicting now, if you allow what they've done remain your fear. No, it does not feel good, so you have to stop the pain by taking the knife out your own heart. You are the one now, which have to say that I have a life to live, and I no longer have to hurt or be angry at myself for those things others did to me.

Why do I say this you ask? I say this because you want acceptance from man and God. God loves you because you are His child, but He hates the things you are doing. God didn't tell the devil to influence that wicked person to hurt you. However, the enemy is influencing you to separate yourself from God's truth. Sin separates us from Him. He did not destroy Sodom and Gomorrah because He hated the people; He destroyed the city because He didn't want that blister of a city to defy His intentions of creating a perfect and happy world. Once a blister bursts, it will spread and affect the part of the body it touches. These people were what the Bible called an evil beast. God made us to be happy but through one man's sin, the only happiness we are going to have is in Jesus Christ, the Savior.

Chapter II

God's Intentions...
"The Other Part"

For the wrath of God is revealed from heaven against all ungodliness and unrighteousness of men, who hold the truth in unrighteousness; Because that which may be none of God is manifest in them; for God hath showed it unto them. For the invisible things of him from the creation of the world are clearly seen, being understood by the things are made, even his eternal power and Godhead; so that they are without excuse: Because that when they knew God, they glorified him not as God, neither were thankful; but became vain in their imaginations, and their foolish heart was darkened. Professing themselves to be wise, they became fools; and the glory of the uncorruptible God into an image made like to be corruptible man, and to birds, and four-footed beasts, and creeping things.

(Romans 1: 20-24 KJV)

an was made in the image of God, but
woman was made from the rib of man to fit
the image of man created by God. People
have taken to their wicked imaginations with ideals that do
not fit. God saw Adam as a man tending to the land and
animals. While looking on him without a mate, as the land
and animals had their pleasure, God decided to give man his
pleasure, so he created woman for Adam. Because of the
flightiness of the mind and heart, man took in his mind to turn
that which was good in the eyes of God into wickedness.

*...Who changed the truth of God into a lie, and worshipped
and served the creature more than the Creator, who is
blessed forever. Amen.* (Romans 1: 25 KJV)

God's beginning and His words cannot be changed. Many
may do as they please, but God sees their actions as filthy
abominations. He hates that He looks on what was not

intended by Him, to be unclean, which man and woman has turned foul.

For this cause God gave them up unto vile affections: for even their women did changed the natural use into that which is against nature: (Romans 1:26 KJV)

A woman was formed to have body parts to please a man; God made these parts for pleasure, while making themselves undefiled in the eyes of God.

And likewise also the men, leaving the natural use of the woman, burned in their own lust one toward another; men with men working that which is unseemly, and receiving in themselves that recompense of their error which was meet. And as they did not like to retain God in their knowledge, God gave them over to a reprobate mind, to do those things which are not convenient;
(Romans 1:27-28 KJV)

It does not matter what translation of the Bible one may read to justify themselves, the same meaning and understanding that we searched for in the beginning will be prevalent and the same. Just because men marry men and women marry women and feel justified in doing so, it is still evil in God's sight. He hates that people have corrupted what He made was to be beautiful. Man has brought evilness on this land by the mind of their doings; and the mind to corrupt others as they are. Also, there are risen churches to not only defy God's ordinances, but publicly announce their shame to the world.

Who knowing the judgement of God, that they which commit such things are worthy of death, not only do the same, but have pleasure in them that do them.

(Romans 1:32)

I read on Facebook where a bitter man stated that people may as well shut up because the courts are on their side and it's going to spread all over the world. The courts with their laws and nearly made bylaws have played a damaging part in this condemned opposition, by allowing men and women the right to display their works of lasciviousness.

If so be that ye have heard him, and have been taught by him, as the truth is in Jesus: That that ye put off concerning the former conversation the old man, which is corrupt according to deceitful lusts; And be renewed in the spirit of your mind. And that ye put on the new man, which after God is created in righteousness and true holiness.

(Ephesians 4:21-24)

If it wasn't for Christ's sake, God would have destroyed this world. He gave Himself to be sacrificed that all might have life, but the abominations of the people of this world are bringing quick deaths and a shortness of life. He could have destroyed us all a long time ago, but He sent redemption to us through sacrificing His life here on earth and through His suffering on the cross.

This world has grown spiritual wheat and tares, which makes it seem like wrong is right, and right is wrong. Many parents have played a huge role in the hurting of this world, by not paying attention to the dealings of their children, and some children were placed in the wrong hands of untrustworthy and treacherous people. Sodom and Gomorrah is another unpleasant momentous, whereby men and women lived an abominable lifestyle with having the spirit of filthy rage, while forcing themselves on innocent people. That place was so corrupt that the wives of Lot were still virgins.

For this ye know, that no whoremonger, nor unclean person, nor covetousness man, who is an idolater, hath any inheritance in the Kingdom of Christ and of God.

(Ephesians 5:5)

Well, one could say that no sin will enter into God's Kingdom, and you are right; however, I believe men being with men and women being with women, God hates more. And the reason many hate this notion is because they are as Sodom and Gomorrah; they do not like to be told the things they cannot do. This is basically the premise; the reason this world is in the shape it is in now. It is extremely sad, but I must be truthful about it.

These doings bring about HIV, AIDS and other deaths that were not intended to be a part of our lives. But through the disobedience of Adam, a door opened to every wrongdoing to be named on this earth. The first thing was death and through that Cain took it upon his heart to kill his brother. Look at fathers and mothers, uncles and aunts; along with sisters and brothers, other relatives committing incest, creating children that will touch other children bringing about a disease that is worse than a spreading fire and will devour like cancer. People have no shame, yet many have God's name in their mouths, but He has no part with them. And that is because of their hate for His word, and He is shamed by their doings being thrown in His face.

But we know that the law is good, if a man use it lawfully: Knowing this, that the law is not made for a righteous man, but for the lawless and disobedient, for the ungodly and for sinners, for unholy and profane, for murderers of fathers and murderers of mothers, for manslayers, For whoremongers, for them that defile themselves with mankind, for menstealers, for liars, for perjured persons, and if there be any other thing that is contrary to sound doctrine; (1Timothy 1:8)

The Bible tells us that, *God so loved the world that he gave his only begotten Son that whosever believeth in him shall not perish but have everlasting life.* God loves us all, but to be a child and a servant of His, one will have to live by every word which proceeds out of the mouth of God. Don't ignore the truth; but read it for yourself, because going against the Word of God will make you a hater of God's Word.

Chapter III

Criminal Acts
The Book of Judges

s it was in the book of Genesis regarding Sodom and Gomorrah, the book of Judges reveals, the criminal doings of the people, the Benjamites. There is a horrific story of how a Levite and his wife wondered into a city named Gibeah to lodge for the night, after leaving his father-in-law's house. While on their way home, night had fallen and they needed an overnight place to stay. The Bible said an old wayfaring man walking in street of that city, saw them, asking where they were going and where they come from. The Levite answered him back letting him know where he was from and that he was on his way to the house of the Lord. The old man encouraged him to board at his house for the night and that he would provide the Levite substance for the evening. And while they were in the house enjoying their meal, when certain men of Belial, the Bible said, of that city surrounded the house. The men began to beat at the door demanding the man of the house to bring the Levite out so they could *know* him. But instead he stepped out and said, "Don't do such a wicked thing, being this man is a visitor in my home", asking them not to commit such an outrageous act. He asked them to take his daughter and the man's concubine, and do as it pleased with them, but to this man do not do such a vile thing. The men wouldn't listen, but the man of that house gave the Levite's wife to those men and they wickedly abuse her all that night. When she walked back to the man's house, she fell dead at the door. The next day her husband found her lying at the threshold and as he motioned her to get up and follow him, he realized she was

dead. He picked her up and took her home and while there,

he cut her body up into twelve pieces, and sent them to all the

coast of Israel. The sight of seeing the woman's body cut into

pieces was so horrible that it made them to say that they had

never seen a deed so horrific since they had come out of

Egypt. Then all the people of Israel assembled in one place

to bring some closure as to how this wicked act (cutting the

woman body into pieces) came about. The Levite told them

his story of how he went to Gibeah and the men of that city

came out at him, to destroy him, and that they forced his

woman all night long, and the end result being her untimely

death. He then went on to explain that he took his wife and

cut her into pieces, and sent her throughout the country to

show how outrageous the men were, while trying to abuse

him, and for the lewdness and folly in Israel.

The head officials came to the conclusion that there would be no rest until this wickedness was brought to justice. They gathered all the tribes together and went among the tribe of Benjamin, asked what evil deeds were being done among them. They told Gibeah to turn those men of Belial over to them so they could put to death. But the people of Benjamin wouldn't hear of it. Instead of turning the men over they arrayed themselves for battle against their own people.

Just as life is today, people rather fight against God rather than to do right. There are so many in this world with that spirit of rebellion, men and women, defying God regarding His Word. One can't change what they are and what they were made to be. God's Word in the beginning of the book of Genesis tells us God created man from the dust of the earth, and after creating man, He saw that man needed a companion, just like He gave animals a mate. He put Adam in a deep sleep the Bible tells us, and created woman Eve from the rib of the man Adam.

If man had the power, which he does not, to change all that is written, he himself would be God's equal, but no man can undo what is already written. Man was made to fit woman, physically, emotionally and spiritually and marriage adorned and patterned after the setting of the Church. Indulging in a renal act is not sex; it is filth in God's eyes because those ways bring about death and sickness. God told man and woman to be fruitful and multiply; one can't be that if they don't have the parts God made in the beginning of life to fulfill those reasons. Belial is having the evil spirit of perverters, and reprobates. Just like the woman was forced upon, children are being forced upon causing them shame and forcing self-hatred on them, which in turns, makes them feel as if they're no good. And because it happened and no one showed them it was wrong, they feel it's the way of life; yet in reality the natural man and woman know that way is wrong, because they fight against the truth.

The Benjamites were completely wiped out of existence, not because they had to be, but because they were given opportunity to turn those evil men in to be judged, but they themselves decided to go into war over something that was wrong. People today are battling over this issue of gay's and lesbians' rights, when in their hearts they know it's wrong. Take a look at the law of justice and you will see the spirit of desolation and abomination having a hold on many in our judicial system. As did the judges back then, the same is happening today. Mind you those that fight against God always lose! We haven't even yet heard from heaven on this matter. Just as in the book of Genesis, Sodom and Gomorrah had the same filthiness infiltrating among them. Angels went into the city to warn that one just man that lived in the city because the entire city had been judged evil. Men rose up in the night and tried to force themselves on men from heaven, while threating to do the same to Lot if he didn't turn those angels over to them. Lot tried to reason with them, just as we are trying to reason. But like back then, people aren't hearing what God is trying to gently cry out. The angels blinded the mob's eyes, and those foolish people went groping about still with the mind to do evil. They all lost their lives because of the spirit of rebellion.

It does not matter what judge allows this filth to infiltrate from city to city, take this and believe, God will deal with the judges and all consenters, along with those that are proud in being and doing these filthy acts where men are being with men and women being with women. We saw this coming also when someone among the Pope said, "Let us let go of the past and forget what has happened." Children lives were forced upon, making them feel like dirt and some took their lives and became addicts, only attempting to stop the brutal touch of the animal that invaded them and stole their innocence. In other words, he was saying shut your eyes to what happened to your children, that this is the way of life which are lies from their father who is Satan. Our heavenly Father is against all such acts and for men of the cloth to say such a thing only shows that he himself is filled with filthy demons. Parents need to watch their children closely and not even trust people in different religious organizations because a lot is going on in many of these places. Find yourself a church where the preacher not just cares about your presence in the church, but cares about your child or children's welfare.

No matter how far one might go to be what they can never be, putting on female garments, getting your body parts removed, or doing anything that would try to persuade yourself that you are that other person, you will have to be able to change the beginning, which can never happen.

Ask ye now, and see whether a man doth travail with child?
Wherefore do I see every man his hand with his hands on
his loins, as a woman in travail,
and all faces are turned into paleness?

(Jeremiah 30:6)

A man does not have a womb, nor does he have a uterus which gives the ability to conceive a child. Man, as I've already written, has different physical parts intended to be used to cause a woman to conceive and bare children. God said be fruitful and multiply and He gave that Word to every living thing that is able to yield offspring of their kind.

And turning the cities of Sodom and Gomorrah into ashes
condemned them with an overthrow, making them an
example unto those that after should live ungodly; (For that
righteous man dwelling among them, in seeing and hearing,
vexed his soul from day to day with their unlawful deeds;)

The Word of God isn't written to please man nor woman; it's written to save men and women, from all the destruction the enemy will bring in the land. But people have chosen to ignore the Word of God by making their own rules and laws. There will be no escaping His judgement. And as it has been said earlier, people aren't geared to being told that they are wrong while being evil. God Himself is saying that He will not tolerate with this kind of insubordination and disobedience. And we need to take a deep look at what is going on in this world today.

Chapter IV

Be Ye Holy, Even as I Am Holy

But he that is joined unto the Lord is one spirit.
(1 Corinthians 6:17)

We know that God speaks for Himself, so howbeit that one being a homosexual claims, that God is using them to spread His Holy Gospel, when they first defy God's Word? God said that the unrighteous (effeminate, or abusers of themselves with mankind) shall not inherit the kingdom of God. Effeminacy and effeminate describes homosexuals and abusers of themselves with mankind and are looked upon by God as Sodomites. So I ask, how can one say God has ordained them to preach His Gospel while indulging in such a wicked nature that the Holy God despises? They are not holy nor are they saved, but just preaching by way of doctrine. I didn't say God couldn't nor did I say He couldn't call them to carry His Gospel, but as their life is now, the Bible has us to know that they are none of His. They may wonder to themselves, "Why is everybody so against us?" But first listen to the Judger of your life, God, who says in 1 Corinthians 5:13, "But them that are without God judgeth. Therefore, PUT AWAY FROM AMONG YOURSELVES THAT WICKED PERSON."

We are not to give consent to this wrong or uphold it. I am not judging them because through the Word of God, we judge ourselves. The righteous warns but never with the heart or mind to harm, kill, or condemn. There is no justification for the lewdness that is spreading like wildfire, and then expect God not to send chastisement on this land we live in. No one is judging them when they see their lifestyles and the burdens these conducts are bringing to this land.

I pray for change that men and women allow God to heal their souls from the bondage that put them apart from God. God does love all of His creation, but He hates the things that has caused His creation hurt, from the time Adam fell and caused death and sin to pollute what He made to be beautiful. The Bible said, "Why call me Lord and do not what I say?" The case scenarios like a good parent that has raised their child or children to do the right thing, but now since they have become adults, they have set standards apart from doing right, when in fact they know they are wrong.

Together the church and society can make a difference. Understanding God's purpose and His plan can bring about a new dawning. His will is for everyone to be shown love by His children. That is how we can defuse Satan's purpose.

Every situation is different and we cannot see all the same. For all that say they love God, there has to be a right now change of heart, especially if you are a man or woman of the cloth, because the Bible clearly says that with loving kindness has He drawn us. No! I did not say excuse or consent to these acts, but our obligation to the Word of God is to love and show love unfeigned. If you can't do this, I am not ashamed to say then you are none of His (God's). In closing, according to Matthew 22:37, it states that Jesus wants us to love the Lord thy God with all thy heart, and all thy soul, and with all thy mind. The second greatest command is to love thy neighbor as thyself.

Scripture References

(All are found in the Holy Bible, King James Version)

1. Page 3, Genesis 4:10
2. Page 5, Philippians 2:5
3. Page 9, Romans 1: 20-24
4. Page 10, Romans 1:26 & 27
5. Page 11, Romans 1:32; Ephesians 4:21-24
6. Page 12, Ephesians 5:5
7. Page 13, 1 Timothy 1:8-10
8. Page 18, Jeremiah 30:6; 2 Peter 2:6, 8 & 9
9. Page 20, 1 Corinthians 6:17; 2 Corinthians 5:13

Meet the Author

allie Carol Rodgers Jones is a mother and a wife for forty-six years. She has a genuine love for God's Word and people. Callie and her husband have a pantry to feed their community and nearby areas. Her heart's desire is to help all who will allow her to; through personal needs and encouragement, specifically children, the elderly and the homeless. She has a passion to help children and teenagers that hang out in the streets because she knows that many of them are there because of broken homes and neglect. If they realize that they have potential to be more than what they present to themselves to be, many of their lives would change. It takes caring people to show them how. As a child, Callie was told that she would never be anybody and that she would never get anywhere in life, but she says, "To God be the glory" for the person she is today. She solely praises God for what He has done and is continuing to do through her life.